Lifemaps

Recovery

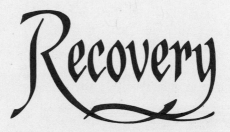

Recovery

When Healing Takes Time

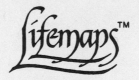

WORD BOOKS
PUBLISHER
WACO, TEXAS

A DIVISION OF
WORD, INCORPORATED

RECOVERY: WHEN HEALING TAKES TIME
Copyright © 1985 by Charles R. Swindoll

Library of Congress Cataloging in Publication Data

Swindoll, Charles R.
  Recovery: when healing takes time.

  (Lifemaps)
  1. Spiritual healing—Biblical teaching. 2. Bible—
Criticism, interpretation, etc. I. Title.
BS680.H4S94 1985   248.8'6   84–27120
ISBN 0–8499–0445–5

Printed in the United States of America

There is an appointed time for everything. And there is a time for every event under heaven—A time to give birth, and a time to die; A time to plant, and a time to uproot what is planted. A time to kill, and a time to heal. . . .

Ecclesiastes 3:1–3

INTRODUCTION

Hippocrates was a Greek physician. He is considered by many to have been "the Father of Medicine." It is he, you may recall, who wrote the immortal Hippocratic Oath still taken by those entering the professional practice of medicine. This ancient physician lived somewhere between 450 B.C. and 375 B.C., which makes him a contemporary of other philosophical thinkers, such as Socrates, Dionysius, Plato, and Aristotle.

Hippocrates wrote much more than the famous oath that bears his name. Other pieces of fine literature flowed from his pen, much of which is still in existence. Most of his works of human wisdom, as we might expect, have to do with the human anatomy, medicine, and healing. It is all interesting reading.

In a piece entitled *Aphorisms,* for example, he wrote: "Extreme remedies are very appropriate for extreme diseases." On another occasion he authored *Precepts.* These words appear in the first chapter: "Healing is a matter of time." While reading those thoughts recently, it occurred to me that one might connect them in a paraphrase that would have a rather significant and relevant ring to it: "Recovering from extreme difficulties usually requires an extreme amount of time."

In our world of "instant" everything, that may not sound very encouraging . . . but it is, more often than not, true. The deeper the wound, the more extensive the damage, the greater amount of time is often needed for us to recover. Wise counsel, Hippocrates! We tend to forget your insightful advice.

Where would the old Greek get such wisdom? His *Aphorisms* and *Precepts* sound almost like the *Proverbs* of Solomon. As a matter of fact, the more you read his writings, the more similar to Solomon they sound.

While entertaining that thought the

other day, I pondered an idea I had never considered before. Hippocrates lived sometime between Solomon the king and Paul the apostle. To fix his existence in biblical history, he lived during the between-the-Testaments era. You may recall that was a four-hundred-year span of time when no Scripture was being written, although the Old Testament books were being compiled. Here's my thought in the form of a question: Could it be that the Greek philosopher, in his research, came across some of Solomon's writings and rephrased a line or two? For example, isn't it possible that something from Solomon's journal (*Ecclesiastes,* by name) could have found its way into the old man's writings?

Consider the first few lines from Ecclesiastes 3:

There is an appointed time for everything. And there is a time for every event under heaven—

A time to give birth, and a time to die;

A time to plant, and a time to uproot what is planted.

A time to kill, and a time to heal;

A time to tear down, and a time to build up (Eccles. 3:1–3).

Tucked away in that third verse is the phrase that intrigues me, ". . . time to heal." Perhaps I am only imagining all this, but I cannot help but wonder if Hippocrates' words, "Healing is a matter of time," might have found their origin in Solomon's statement. We may never know for sure. In any event, the statement remains sound, both medically and biblically. More often than not, healing takes time. And, I repeat, the greater the disease or damage, the more extensive the time to heal.

I have been concerned about this issue for a long, long time. In twenty-five years of ministry I have had a great deal of contact with people who hurt. Their pain has come from every conceivable source. Those who have seemed most disillusioned have been the ones who anticipated but did not experience quick recovery. Many of them were promised such by people who held out the hope of a "miracle." When the alleged divine intervention did not transpire, their anguish reached the breaking point. I have looked into their faces and heard their cries. I have witnessed their response—everything from quiet disappointment to bitter, cursing cynicism . . . from tearful sadness to violent acts of suicide. Most have been sincere, intelligent, Christian people.

Many other ministers, it seems, enjoy the role of leading people into rather rapid relief of their pain. Admittedly, I could easily envy such a joyful and popular ministry. More often than not, it seems my lot to help those who do not "heal in a hurry," no matter how hard they try, no matter how firmly they believe, no matter how sincerely they pray. Even though I would love to perform instant miracles (or at least promise recovery "within a week or two"), I am not able to do so. Maybe that is the reason I am so intrigued with the combined thoughts of Hippocrates and Solomon. Since I deal constantly with people in pain, I am left to search for answers that make sense, even though they will never make the headlines.

This is a book about the answers I have found. I have no cure-all solutions to offer, no secret formula that will have you on your feet, smiling, in twenty-four hours. I wish I did, but I don't. I do have some things to say, however, that may give you fresh hope and renewed perspective in the recovery process. It will not come from some philosophical meanderings or superstious hocus-pocus.

Everything I have to say finds its origin in Scripture, God's unfailing, ever-reliable Book of truth. If you are weary of the sensational, if the get-well-quick answers haven't worked for you, if it seems that the miracles of overnight relief are for someone else, then perhaps this book is for you.

I wish I could guarantee you healing simply as a result of your reading these pages. I cannot. But I can promise you this: A heart that understands, truth that will not leave you in the lurch or disillusioned, and a God who cares . . . whose plan is unsearchable, whose ways are unfathomable, whose counsel is dependable.

Chuck Swindoll
Fullerton, California

TIME TO HEAL

I have seen a lot of bumper stickers that read:

I'D RATHER BE SAILING.

But I have never seen one that reads,

I'D RATHER BE SHIPWRECKED!

I doubt I ever will. Sailing across the water is an exhilarating, ecstatic experience, but sinking under the water is nothing short of terrifying, especially if the sea is rough and the winds are stormy.

Having spent over a month on the ocean during my days in the Marine Corps, I have had my share of high waves and maddening windstorms. On one occasion the swells were somewhere between thirty and forty feet high and no one—not even the skipper—thought we would ever see land again. Talk about feeling helpless! Going through such life-threatening situations gives one an absolutely realistic perspective on and respect for the sea. I never see a large ocean-going vessel without having a flashback to my days on the Pacific. How different from what I expected! Instead of an uninterrupted calm, relaxed voyage in the buoyant waters of the deep, my whole world was turned topsy-turvy. Every time I hear some novice speak glibly about how much fun it would be to sail a little boat across the seas, I shudder down inside. What we expect is seldom what we experience.

This came home to me in a fresh way some time ago when I read about the twenty-year reunion of most of those who were involved in the formation of the old American Football League. The seasoned sports veterans and owners swapped stories and enjoyed a full evening of laughs and reflections together. Among those present back then was Al Davis, currently the owner of the Los Angeles Raiders. He remembers that all those sitting at his table stared with envy at Nicky Hilton, who was to speak on that eventful evening in 1959. Everyone's feelings of expectation back then were only heightened when the man was introduced as having recently made $100,000 in the baseball business in the city of Los Angeles.

Mr. Hilton stood to his feet as the place broke into thunderous applause. He stepped to the microphone and said he needed to correct what had been said. It was not he who'd had that experience, it was his brother Baron. And it wasn't at Los Angeles, but San Diego. And it wasn't baseball, it was football. And it wasn't $100,000, it was $1 million . . . and he didn't make it, he *lost* it!

It's amazing what you discover when you look beneath the surface, isn't it? Realism always takes the wind out of idealism's sails.

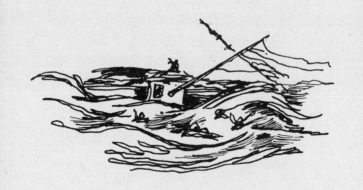

HISTORICAL INTERRUPTION

That's exactly what happened to a man named Paul, who lived in the days of the first century. For years he had one great dream: to go to Rome, the capital of the Empire. The driving force of his life was to have an audience with the Caesar (Nero) and, eyeball-to-eyeball, present to him the claims of Jesus Christ.

A Dream Becomes a Nightmare

Not a bad idea! Sounds like a worthy objective, a dream . . . and when you consider that getting there called for a lengthy trip aboard ship from Palestine to Italy, you could almost envision a Mediterranean cruise to boot. But it wasn't a cruise; it was a disaster. The ship didn't sail; it sank. And he didn't arrive immediately in Italy; he landed fifty miles south of Sicily. And it wasn't the splendid metropolis of Rome; it was the rugged island named Malta.

What a disappointment! Picture in your mind the fierce storm and the panic that must have accompanied those who escaped with their lives:

And all of us in the ship were two hundred and seventy-six persons. And when they had eaten enough, they began to lighten the ship by throwing out the wheat into the sea. And when day came, they could not recognize the land; but they did observe a certain bay with a beach, and they resolved to drive the ship onto it if they could. And casting off the anchors, they left them in the sea while at the same time they were loosening the ropes of the rudders, and hoisting the foresail to the wind, they were heading for the beach. But striking a reef where two seas met, they ran the vessel aground; and the prow stuck fast and remained immovable, but the stern began to be broken up by the force of the waves. And the soldiers' plan was to kill the prisoners, that none of them

should swim away and escape; but the
centurion, wanting to bring Paul safely
through, kept them from their intention, and
commanded that those who could swim
should jump overboard first and get to land,
and the rest should follow, some on planks,
and others on various things from the ship.
And thus it happened that they all were
brought safely to land (Acts 27:37–44).

All 276 swam, gagged, gasped,
struggled, then finally sloshed ashore,
safe yet soaked, and exhausted. It was
an unexpected, tumultuous, distant
detour. So it is when you find yourself
dumped on an island named Malta when
all along you had Italy in your sights and
the dream of Rome on your heart.

The Beginning of Recovery

If I may interrupt the story, allow me
a few moments to add a practical
dimension that is easily overlooked.

Those who are victims need what places like Malta can provide. It may seem to be a barren, lonely, desperate spot, but its therapy is solitude and in its quiet, gentle breezes are renewal, refreshment, and healing. In a word, I'm referring to *recovery* . . . which, I remind you, takes time.

May I go deeper? God plans our Maltas. These transitional islands may seem forlorn and fearsome. This opinion is intensified if you arrive there on the edge of despair, suffering from a neurotic drive to accomplish more, more, more. Those who opt for burning out en route to Rome fear rusting out at Malta, but that doesn't occur. On the contrary, it takes Malta to show us how to stop just existing and start living again. What appears as nothing more than the death of a dream is, in actuality, the first step in the process of recovery.

As any student of the New Testament would tell you, Paul's life over the previous twelve to fifteen months had been anything but serene. He had appeared before several frowning judges in one courtroom scene after another. He had experienced mob violence, physical abuse, demonic and satanic oppression, imprisonment, the pain of misunderstanding by friend and foe alike, and more than one threat on his life. Most of those things he endured alone . . . so toss in the loneliness factor. The storm at sea was a fitting and climactic analogy for those long months prior to the shipwreck off the coast of Malta. Forgive me if I sound uncaring, but it took a shipwreck to jolt Paul's perspective back into focus. The disaster at sea followed by the forced change of pace on Malta was precisely what he needed for the process of recuperation and repair to begin.

Sir Winston Churchill, the late prime minister of England, was a leader I have admired for many years. Through intense years of political pressure, heightened by his country's devastating war with Nazi Germany, Churchill maintained a remarkable sense of balance. His wisdom and wit remained intact and panic never seemed to drain his inner reservoir of confident hope. I have studied his life with keen curiosity. He once wrote a brief essay entitled "Painting as a Pastime" in which he unveiled his secret of sustaining such a peaceful mindset. It is worth our careful attention.

Many remedies are suggested for the avoidance of worry and mental overstrain by persons who, over prolonged periods, have to bear exceptional responsibilities and discharge duties upon a very large scale. Some advise exercise, and others, repose. Some counsel travel, and others retreat. Some praise solitude, and others, gaiety. No doubt all these may play their part according to the individual temperament. But the element which is constant and common in all of them is Change.

Change is the master key. A man can wear out a particular part of his mind by continually using it and tiring it, just in the same way as he can wear out the elbows of his coat. There is, however, this difference between the living cells of the brain and inanimate articles: One cannot mend the frayed elbows of a coat by rubbing the sleeves or shoulders; but the tired parts of the mind can be rested and strengthened, not merely by rest, but by using other parts. It is not enough merely to switch off the lights which play upon the main and ordinary field of interest; a new field of interest must be illuminated. It is no use saying to the tired mental muscles—if one may coin such an expression—"I will give you a good rest." "I will go for a long walk," or "I will lie down and think of nothing." The mind keeps busy just the same. If it has been weighing and measuring, it goes on weighing and measuring. If it has been worrying, it goes on worrying. It is only when new cells are called into activity, when new stars become the lords of the ascendant, that relief, repose, refreshment are afforded.

A gifted American psychologist has said, "Worry is a spasm of the emotion; the mind catches hold of something and will not let it go." It is useless to argue with the mind in this condition. The stronger the will, the more futile the task. One can only gently insinuate something else into its convulsive grasp. And if this something else is rightly chosen, if it is really attended by the illumination of another field of interest, gradually, and often quite swiftly, the old undue grip relaxes and the process of recuperation and repair begins. . .[1]

Lest you think that "doing nothing" is all that is involved in one's stopover at Malta, Churchill's counsel has been mentioned here. Paul does not merely walk along the beach and finger a few seashells . . . nor does he spend weeks staring at sunsets, wiggling his toes in the sand. For him to heal, change was needed, not simply stoic silence.

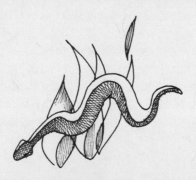

PERSONAL TREATMENT

Dr. Luke, the writer of the Acts narrative, mentions a couple of the incidents that transpired between Paul and the island natives. The New English Bible refers to these people as "rough islanders," implying that they had limited education and were driven by superstitious beliefs, which is seen in the account we're about to examine.

Extraordinary Kindness

And the natives showed us extraordinary kindness; for because of the rain that had set in and because of the cold, they kindled a fire and received us all. But when Paul had gathered a bundle of sticks and laid them on the fire, a viper came out because of the heat, and fastened on his hand. And when the natives saw the creature hanging from his hand, they began saying to one another, "Undoubtedly this man is a murderer, and though he has been saved from the sea, justice has not allowed him to live" (Acts 28:2–4).

Initially, the shipwreck victims were greeted with extraordinary kindness. An early winter rainstorm drenched the island and left everyone shivering because of the cold. Unusually hospitable, the islanders built a large fire and treated the visitors with a marked degree of kindness.

Suddenly, the scene changes.

Unjust Criticism

Aroused and angered by the fire, a viper crawled out of the stack of timber and attached itself to Paul's hand. Its bite was so deep and penetrating that Paul was unable to shake his hand free from the snake. As this was being witnessed by the natives, they jumped to a conclusion that was both cruel and inaccurate. They were suddenly convinced that Paul's calamity was proof of guilt.

Interestingly, even though these barbarians (the actual Greek term translated "natives") lacked education and refined culture, they had an inner standard of justice. Their opinion, however incorrect, was an instantaneous one: "Undoubtedly this man is a murderer." To them the snake bite represented justice having her due.

There is something amazingly relevant about this episode. A "punishment" mindset is not limited to rough islanders in the Mediterannean. Heathen tribespeople aren't the only ones who jump to the erroneous conclusion that those who suffer are simply getting what they deserve. Justified punishment—"calamity is proof of guilt." Abominable theology!

The classic case in Scripture is Job.

Here was an upright man who had worked hard, dealt honestly with people, reared a fine family, and walked with his God. Then suddenly, seemingly out of nowhere, a whirlwind of multiple tragedies drove the man to his knees. It was bad enough to lose his livestock and all other means of income, but on top of that he lost each one of his children and finally his health. With hardly a moment between these calamities to catch his breath and gain a measure of equilibrium, Job was reduced to a painful hulk of humanity, covered from head to toe with oozing skin ulcers.

Exit: compassion.

Enter: thoughtless counselors of blame. One man after another pointed a long bony finger into the face of the sufferer, frowning at him with condemning words and advising him to confess his guilt. In effect, each one said, "You're getting what you deserve." The confrontational dialogue contained in the ancient Book of Job is remarkably relevant. Who knows? Maybe it flashed across Paul's mind when he heard, "Undoubtedly, this man is a murderer . . . justice has not allowed him to live!"

I wish there were some way for sufferers to be delivered from such unjust and unfair criticism, but I know of none. It is painful enough to endure the severe blows of life . . . but when words of condemnation coming from superstition and prejudice bite into us, causing the venom of guilt to spread and poison our minds, it is almost more than we can bear.

Inappropriate Exaltation

Quickly, however, Paul shook off the viper. As it fell into the fire, leaving Paul free from any ill effects, the natives' eyes grew large with amazement. They waited and waited for Paul to drop dead. When he didn't, when they witnessed his resilience, ". . . they changed their minds and began to say that he was a god."

I cannot help but smile when I read this abrupt change of opinion. First the man is a murderer, now he's a god. When calamity struck, he was getting his due—punishment by death. But once he recovered, he is suddenly catapulted to the superhuman realm, and they are ready to worship him.

A. T. Robertson, New Testament scholar of yesteryear, recalls Paul's similar experience in reverse many years before this encounter on Malta. That one occurred in a city named Lystra, where Paul was first elevated to the place of a god, Mercury, only to be stoned shortly thereafter by the very same people who had earlier deified him. With seasoned wisdom, Dr. Robertson adds this biting comment, "So fickle is popular favor." [2]

I cannot let this pass without a personal comment to you who read this book. It is quite possible that your

situation today has been intensified by
a similar reversal of opinion against you.
You once knew success. You had the
respect of others. You were in demand:
a competent, admired, highly honored
individual who drank daily from the well
of fresh praise . . . right? How things
have changed! You now find yourself
"shelved" and virtually passed by,
perhaps even hated by a few. Your world
has suffered a head-on collision and
you're bloody from having gone through
the windshield of reversed reputation.
Those who once quoted you now
criticize you. "So fickle is popular favor."
Full recovery, I remind you, calls for a
healing that will take time. And it cannot
occur, unfortunately, without some scars
remaining. The two scars you will have
to deal with the most are
disillusionment, which comes from
sudden deflation, and bitterness, the
result of prolonged blame.

RELATIONAL CONCERN

Now, back to our story on Malta. The writer includes a couple of vignettes from the island that speak with relevance to us today.

Now in the neighborhood of that place were lands belonging to the leading man of the island, named Publius, who welcomed us and entertained us courteously three days. And it came about that the father of Publius was lying in bed afflicted with recurrent fever and dysentery; and Paul went in to see him and after he had prayed, he laid his hands on him and healed him. And after this had happened, the rest of the people on the island who had diseases were coming to him and getting cured. And they also honored us with many marks of respect; and when we were setting sail, they supplied us with all we needed (Acts 28:7–10).

It may seem a technical point to mention, but take a moment to notice the repeated pronouns "us" and "we." The writer of the narrative is obviously including himself. Who is he? Luke. And what is his profession? Physician. My point is this. Here is a physician, an educated, well-trained medical doctor whose expertise is the diagnosis of disease—in this case, "recurrent fever and dysentery" which caused Publius' father to be bedridden. Dr. Luke could diagnose the ailment, but he was at a loss to bring about a cure. Interestingly, Paul was not a trained, professional physician, but he possessed the supernatural, God-given ability to do what Luke could not do.

Instant Healing

Initially, Dr. Luke stood back as God worked through His servant Paul who, after praying for the aging victim, "laid his hands on him and healed him." The word originally used by the physician-writer is *iaomai,* a Greek term that refers, more often than not, to instantaneous healing. An on-the-spot miracle. Paul, please understand, was not the source of such power, only the vehicle . . . the human instrument through whom God supernaturally worked.

I am as impressed with Dr. Luke's lack of envy as I am with the apostle Paul's spiritual gift. The physician stepped aside. Although we may be certain his medical training had left him no room for divine miracles, his theology did! Without a moment's hesitation the professional was willing to stand back and watch God do the unusual.

And that last word is worth repeating for emphasis—an on-the-spot miracle is *unusual*, an exception to the general rule. For too long people have been led to believe that virtually in every case they can "expect a miracle." And to make matters worse, when the miracle doesn't occur, they are told that something is wrong with them, they are harboring sin, they are not strong enough in their faith . . . on and on. I shall restrain myself from grinding an axe at this point, but I must state that there are few areas in which there is greater confusion than this concept of instant healing. Sufferers are being promised miracles by many alleged authorities—some are sincere, some naive, some professional con artists—and when the miracle does not come, the damage done is always tragic and occasionally irreparable.

Let's understand that there are times when God does indeed heal . . . instantly, miraculously, unexplainably. I repeat, such miracles are rare—unusual exceptions to the rule—and they remind us that the One who made us certainly has the power over our physical bodies. More on that later.

Prolonged Recovery

Look again at the last part of this account:

And after this had happened, the rest of the people on the island who had diseases were coming to him and getting cured. And they also honored us with many marks of respect; and when we were setting sail, they supplied us with all we needed (Acts 28:9–10).

As the word of that miracle traveled across the island, the rest of those with ailments came for healing. A cursory reading of what occurred could leave us with the impression that everyone who came received a similar instantaneous miracle. Not so. The original term used by Dr. Luke to describe the people's being "cured" is altogether different from the one he used for Publius's father. This word is *therapeuō*, from which we get our English word, "therapy." One reputable source writes that:

. . . it might better be translated . . . *were treated*. It suggests not miraculous healings but medical treatment, probably at the hands of Luke the physician. Verses 10 and

11 suggest that this medical ministry lasted throughout the three months stay at Malta. . . .[3]

In other words, these people went through a process, a prolonged period of recovery, which lasted perhaps for three months—maybe longer. If Luke were involved with Paul, this would be one of the earliest references in all of Scripture to "overseas medical missionary" work.

Sometimes, healing is instantaneous—*iaomai* recovery. More often than not, it takes time to heal—*therâpeuō* recovery, under the care and watchful eyes of a competent physician.

PRACTICAL LESSONS

We seldom think in terms of the lessons to be learned or the benefits connected to prolonged recovery. As I mentioned earlier, we like quick turn-arounds, instant changes from sickness to health. We much prefer hearing accounts of miracles as opposed to long, nonsensational stories of slow recoveries. In fact, we tend to be impatient with those who can't seem to take our advice and "snap out of it" or "get well soon," like the greeting card urges them to do. But like it or not, more often than not, the wise words of Hippocrates are true: "Healing is a matter of time."

Respect . . . Rather than Resentment

The one who needs time to heal, the individual who requires several months—perhaps, several years—to heal, is often the recipient of resentment. This works against the recovery process. Instead of being affirmed and encouraged to press on through the pain, allowing oneself sufficient time to get back on stream, the sufferer encounters resentment and impatience. Uninvited advice that lacks understanding and reveals disrespect begins to flow. The result is predictable.

This is especially true of those who must climb out of a background of emotional trauma. It took years for the damage to be done, yet many expect overnight recovery. For some there is the added stigma of attempted suicide or time spent in a psychiatric ward or mental hospital. For some, their past has been strewn with the litter of a prison experience, a divorce, a rape, child abuse, or some other ego-shattering blow on their self-esteem. No one on the face of the earth would love to be healed and back in the mainstream of life more than these strugglers, but for them the therapy is a prolonged and painful process, not an instant miracle.

My plea on their behalf is that we love and respect them rather than resent them. Some, I realize, may go to the extreme, play on our sympathy, and take advantage of our compassion. But more often than not, however, those who are recovering want nothing more than to be well, whole, responsible, functioning adults who carry their share of the load. Just as it is possible to hurry the very young through childhood, not giving them the benefit of growing up slowly and securely, so it is possible to hurry the very ill through recovery, robbing them of the benefits of healing slowly and permanently.

May I ask a favor? Please read that sentence again, with feeling.

Wisdom . . . Not Just Knowledge

I have said a lot to those who deal with the hurting, but not much to the sufferer personally. Let me speak to you for a moment.

A major benefit of taking time to heal occurs within you. Almost imperceptibly, you are becoming a person with keener sensitivity, a broader base of understanding, and a longer fuse! Patience is a by-product of pain. So is tolerance with others and obedience before God. It is difficult to know how to classify these characteristics, but for lack of a better title, let's call the whole package *wisdom*.

For too many years in your life you have operated strictly on the basis of knowledge . . . human absorption of facts and natural reaction to others. But affliction has now entered your life, and even though you would much prefer to have it over with, it has not ended. Difficult though it may be for you to believe it, the pain you are forced to endure is reshaping and remaking you deep within.

It is as David, the psalmist, once wrote:

Before I was afflicted I went astray, But now I keep Thy word. It is good for me that I was afflicted, that I may learn Thy statutes. I know, O Lord, that Thy judgments are righteous, and that in faithfulness Thou hast afflicted me (Psalm 119:67, 71, 75).

A quick glance back over those words is worthwhile. David admits that a much greater desire to obey (v. 67), a much-more-teachable spirit (v. 71), and a much-less-arrogant attitude (v. 75) were now his to claim, thanks to prolonged affliction.

Human knowledge comes naturally. It is enhanced by schooling and it is enlarged by travel. But with it there often comes carnal pride, a sense of self-sufficiency, and tough independence. This kind of knowledge can cause us to become increasingly less interested in the spiritual dimension of life. As our reservoir of horizontal knowledge grows, our skin gets thicker and often our inner being (called "the heart" in Scripture) becomes calloused. Then comes pain. Some physical ailment levels us to mere mortality. Or an emotional collapse. A domestic conflict explodes and we are reduced to a cut above zero. The affliction (whatever it may be) paralyzes our productivity and we are cast adrift in a sea of private turmoil and, possibly, public embarrassment. And to make matters worse, we are convinced we'll never, ever recover.

At just such a dead-end street, divine wisdom waits to be embraced. She brings with her a beautiful blend of insight— the kind we never had with all our knowledge—genuine humility, a perception of others, and an incredible sensitivity toward God. Stop and think. Without this prolonged period of recovery, such God-given wisdom may very well pass you by. During the time it is taking you to heal, wisdom is replacing knowledge. The vertical dimension is coming into clearer focus.

Balance . . . Freedom from Extremes

If you'll allow me yet another comment on the benefits of taking time to heal, I cannot ignore the value of balance. It has been my own experience as well as my observation of others that a lengthy recovery time rivets into our heads the importance of bringing our lives back from the fringes of the extreme. And I especially have in mind either the extreme of *too much work,* where our world is too structured, too product-oriented, too intense and responsible (to the point of neurosis) or *too little work,* where irresponsibility, inactivity, and indifference have marked our paths. During the recovery stage, it is amazing how God enables us to see the foolish extremes of our former lives.

Eugene Peterson, in a work entitled *A Long Obedience in the Same Direction,* says what I am trying to describe as he compares Western and Eastern cultures:

The Christian has to find a better way to avoid the sin of Babel than by imitating the lilies of the field, who "neither toil nor spin." The pretentious work which became Babel and its pious opposite which developed at Thessalonica are displayed today on the broad canvasses of Western and Eastern cultures respectively.

Western culture takes up where Babel left off and deifies human effort as such. The machine is the symbol of this way of life that attempts to control and manage. Technology promises to give us control over the earth and over other people. But the promise is not fulfilled: lethal automobiles, ugly buildings and ponderous bureaucracies ravage the earth and empty lives of meaning. Structures become more important than the people who live in them. Machines become more important than the people who use them. We care more for our possessions with which we hope to make our way in the world than for our thoughts and dreams which tell us who we are in the world.

Eastern culture, on the other hand, is a variation on the Thessalonican view. There is a deep-rooted pessimism regarding human effort. Since all work is tainted with selfishness and pride, the solution is to withdraw from all activity into pure being. The symbol of such an attitude is the Buddha—an enormous fat person sitting cross-legged, looking at his own navel. Motionless, inert, quiet. All trouble comes from doing too much; therefore, do nothing. Step out of the rat race. The world of motion is evil, so quit doing everything. Say as little as possible; do as little as possible; finally, at the point of perfection, you will say nothing and do nothing. The goal is to withdraw absolutely and finally from action, from thought, from passion.

The two cultures are in collision today and many think that we must choose between them.[4]

As a result of this tendency toward extremes, many people break, and the inner destruction leaves them in shambles. It takes time to reorder and balance out our personal lives.

THEOLOGICAL EXPLANATION

Normally, in a book of this nature, I would quietly conclude my thoughts and shy away from getting very deep into theology. Primarily, because I am not writing to people who are trained to think in theological terms. Secondly, because I haven't the space to do a thorough enough job to satisfy the few who desire that I plumb the depths of the theology of healing. But my conscience will not allow me to conclude these pages without at least attempting to hit the high points and, hopefully, bring some light from God and His inerrant Word into a room that has been made darker by man and his erroneous opinion. People in pain suffer enough dealing with the truth . . . but to make them suffer even more, crushed by the brutal blows of error, is cruel and unjust punishment.

Therefore, please consider these final pages with an open mind. They are original ideas that have come to me through no other source than the Scriptures. They help me think through my position on healing and they offer an explanation to those who ask why and why not. Although theological in nature, my suggestions are worded in such a way that you do not need a seminary degree to understand them.

Five Physical Facts

You've heard of the four spiritual laws. Here are five physical facts . . . not nearly as popular, but they are equally important.

Fact One: There are two types of sin: original and personal. *Original sin* is traced back to Adam and Eve, the first humans, and their fall in the Garden of Eden. That act of disobedience contaminated the entire human race, leaving all mankind spiritually dead and distant from God.

Therefore, just as through one man sin entered into the world, and death through sin, and so death spread to all men, because all sinned (Rom. 5:12).

Personal sin is an individual matter. When we disobey, when each one of us chooses to transgress God's will, we commit personal sin and we suffer the consequences. Because we are sinful by nature (original sin), we are sinners by choice (personal sin).

For all have sinned and fall short of the glory of God (Rom. 3:23).

Fact Two: Original sin introduced sickness, suffering, and death into the human race.

Because of the Adamic fall, mankind

must live with, struggle through, and accept the "fallout" of original sin. In the broadest sense of the word, all sickness is the result of *original* sin. In the same way we could say all auto accidents are the result of human weakness.

> . . . The soul who sins will die (Ezek. 18:4b).
> For since by a man [Adam] came death. . . . For as in Adam all die . . . (1 Cor. 15:21a, 22a).

Fact Three: Often there exists a direct relationship between personal sin and physical sickness.

There are numerous examples in Scripture, as well as in life, where someone became ill because that person acted in disobedience.

King David, for example:

> When I kept silent about my sin, my body wasted away through my groaning all day

long. For day and night Thy hand was heavy upon me; my vitality was drained away as with the fever-heat of summer. [Selah.] I acknowledged my sin to Thee, and my iniquity I did not hide (Psalm 32:3–5).

The man whom Jesus healed:

Afterward Jesus found him in the temple, and said to him, "Behold, you have become well, do not sin any more, so that nothing worse may befall you" (John 5:14).

The carnal Corinthians:

For this reason many among you are weak and sick, and a number sleep ("sleep," in this case, meant "dead") (1 Cor. 11:30).

In such cases, confession of sin is the first step toward healing.

Fact Four: Sometimes there is *no* relation between personal sin and physical sickness.

One's illness cannot always be traced back to an act of disobedience. Sometimes our suffering lacks any connection with our own transgression. The man born blind, for example:

And as He passed by, He saw a man blind from birth. And His disciples asked Him, saying, "Rabbi, who sinned, this man or his parents, that he should be born blind?" Jesus answered, "It was neither that this man sinned, nor his parents, but it was in order that the works of God might be displayed in him (John 9:1–3).

In Hebrews 4:15 we read that Jesus sympathizes with us in our weaknesses. If all such infirmities were traceable to sin, rather than being the recipients of our Lord's sympathy, we would be challenged to repent, to confess. Furthermore, upon confession, our every sickness would be instantly healed . . . if personal sin and physical sickness were inseparably linked.

Fact Five: It is not God's will that everyone be healed in this life.

Please continue reading with an open mind. And continue to think theologically, not emotionally or traditionally.

There are specific cases in Scripture where godly, dedicated, and spiritually pure men remained victims of disease and weakness—Epaphroditus (Phil. 2:27) and Trophimus (1 Tim. 4:20), for example. Even the great apostle Paul prayed on three separate occasions for the removal of "a thorn in the flesh," which hindered his being free of pain. Yet the thorn remained with him. Although it was not God's will that he be healed, the man learned numerous and valuable lessons as a result of the pain and affliction.

And because of the surpassing greatness of the revelations, for this reason, to keep me from exalting myself, there was given me a thorn in the flesh, a messenger of Satan to buffet me—to keep me from exalting myself! Concerning this I entreated the Lord three times that it might depart from me. And He has said to me, "My grace is sufficient for you, for power is perfected in weakness." Most gladly, therefore, I will rather boast about my weaknesses, that the power of Christ may dwell in me. Therefore I am well content with weaknesses, with insults, with distresses, with persecutions, with difficulties, for Christ's sake; for when I am weak, then I am strong (2 Cor. 12:7–10).

There are many who teach that there is "healing in the atonement." By this they mean that the one who believes in Jesus Christ's atoning death for sin not only receives deliverance from sin but also deliverance from sin's by-products, sickness and disease. They base this teaching on Isaiah 53:5, a verse of Scripture that appears in a passage predicting Messiah's death. Allow me to state the verse in its surrounding context.

Surely our griefs He Himself bore, and our sorrows He carried; yet we ourselves esteemed Him stricken, smitten of God, and afflicted. But he was pierced through for our transgressions, He was crushed for our iniquities; the chastening for our well-being fell upon Him, and by His scourging we are healed. All of us like sheep have gone astray, each of us has turned to his own way; but the Lord has caused the iniquity of us all to fall on Him.

He was oppressed and He was afflicted, yet He did not open His mouth; like a lamb that is led to slaughter, and like a sheep that is silent before its shearers, so He did not open His mouth (Isa. 53:4–7).

A close and careful look at the prophet's words will reveal that the context is one of great physical pain which Messiah would endure on the cross. But the point is, His suffering is for our spiritual benefit. The subject being dealt with is the sinner's "transgressions," our "iniquities." The death of Messiah provides the solution to our spiritual deadness. Our sins are forgiven because He once for all cleansed us when He was crucified. Hence, by His physical death we are granted spiritual healing. I agree, there *is* healing in the atonement . . . spiritual healing from the sins that kept us from God, healing from the overcoming power and influence of our adversary, healing from the grave that once frightened us, and healing from death that would otherwise conquer us.

And, of course, God promises to heal us of all illness and affliction once we pass from this life into glory. Such instant healing is part of the "eternal package" we receive when these bodies "put on immortality" (1 Cor. 15:53). But lest you think I am saying God never instantly heals anyone on this earth, I must clarify and restate my position. I certainly do believe in divine healing, but I do not believe in divine heal*ers,* as we see them in action today. On several occasions in my ministry, I have seen our Lord sovereignly step onto the scene of suffering and instantly bring healing. Neither time nor space allow me to describe these eventful moments. But there was no doubt that God (and He alone) chose to overrule the course of nature and remove the sickness or break the fever or dissolve the cancerous tumor or reverse the direction of an otherwise terminal disease. But in none of those cases was any human agency responsible for the miracle . . . only God.

All that any of us could do was pray—*and pray we did!* Fervently, confidently, believingly, faithfully we prayed. The attending physician also did all that could be done. And divine healing occurred. Sometimes it was the result of the sick person's confession of sin—since there was a relation between sin and sickness as I described in the third fact above. This seems to be the case in James 5:14–16.

Is anyone among you sick? Let him call for the elders of the church and let them pray over him, anointing him with oil in the name of the Lord; and the prayer offered in faith will restore the one who is sick and the Lord will raise him up, and if he has committed sins, they will be forgiven him. Therefore, confess your sins to one another, and pray for one another, so that you may be healed. The effective prayer of a righteous man can accomplish much.

At other times the healing came for no explainable or logical reason. God simply and sovereignly chose to bring relief. And we praised His name.

But more often than not, I must confess, as I did at the beginning of this book, healing has taken time. Recovery has been a difficult, painful process . . . but certainly not without its own benefits, which I have attempted to describe.

CONCLUSION

There are three general responses to a book on this subject. First, it is possible that you have read my words and kept an open mind to my thinking, yet you honestly disagree with what I have presented. You are convinced that God works in a different way than I have described and that miracles are the rule, not the exception. I appreciate your open-minded attention, and I respect your right to disagree. Please be assured of this—there are difficulties to be wrestled with, no matter which "side" we may take. My prayer is that God will comfort and encourage you as you trust Him to intervene. If He does, I will rejoice with you. If He does not, I hope you will not become disillusioned, confused, and bitter, as have so many I have dealt with who approached their suffering from that perspective.

Second, you may find yourself encouraged and relieved because these things make sense. You agree, more often than not, it takes time to heal. And you are affirmed in the recovery process. Perhaps you were getting anxious and jumping to some false conclusions, misreading God's silence and failing to glean His wisdom. You have decided to rest rather than strive. I am sincerely grateful that you have "hung tough" as my teenagers say. Your renewed determination to learn and to grow through these stretching days will be *abundantly* rewarded. The roots grow deep when the winds are strong. Working through is always—always— more painful than walking out. But in the end, ah, what confident honesty, what calm assurance, what character depth!

Third, you may still be making up your mind. Some of this sounds reasonable. You identify and agree with several of the issues I have raised, but in the final analysis you're not ready to come down with both feet and say, "Yes, that's where I stand." You may be pleased (and surprised) to know that I consider this an intelligent response. The subject of pain is a profound one. The process involved in working through some of these issues is intensely difficult, sometimes terribly complex. I may be able to address them in these few pages, but, believe me, in no way have I mastered the message I proclaim. How all these things fit together into God's perfect plan, I am not anywhere near prepared to say. Why human evil and its consequences are allowed such green lights by a holy God is another baffling paradox. I agree with Scott Peck:

I have not learned all about human evil; I am learning. In fact, I am just beginning to learn. . . . Do not regard anything written here as the last word. Indeed, the purpose of the book is to lead us to dissatisfaction with our current state of ignorance of the subject.[5]

So my counsel to all, no matter how you respond to my book, is that you join me in continuing to search for answers. Let's listen to the wisdom of the Scriptures. Let's pay close attention to the "still small voice" of God who whispers to us in our pleasure and shouts to us in our pain (C. S. Lewis). And most of all, let's not allow a few technical definitions or theological differences to push us apart. There are many more things that draw us together than there are that separate us. We still need each other.

It is difficult enough to handle life when we stand together. But doing battle with one another in addition to struggling through our shipwrecks, our Maltas, our storms, and our thorns can be almost unbearable. We need all the support we can get during recovery. As we take time to heal, let's also take time to hear . . . to care . . . to accept . . . to affirm . . . to pray . . . to say, "I love you. I am with you, no matter how much time it takes for you to heal."

NOTES

1. Winston S. Churchill, "Painting as a Pastime," an essay from the book *A Man of Destiny* compiled by the editors of Country Beautiful (Waukesha, WI: Country Beautiful Foundation, Inc., 1965), p. 63.

2. Archibald Thomas Robertson, *Word Pictures in the New Testament*, Vol. III, The Acts of the Apostles (Nashville, TN: Broadman Press, 1930), p. 480.

3. Everett F. Harrison, ed. *The Wycliffe Bible Commentary* (Chicago, IL: Moody Press, 1962), p. 1176.

4. Taken from *A Long Obedience in*

the Same Direction by Eugene H.
Peterson, © 1980 by Inter-Varsity
Christian Fellowship of the USA and
used by permission of Inter Varsity
Press, Downers Grove, IL 60515 (pp.
102, 103).

5. M. Scott Peck, *People of the Lie*
(New York, NY: Simon and Schuster,
1983), p. 10.

ABOUT THE AUTHOR

Ordained into the gospel ministry in 1963, Dr. Charles R. Swindoll has developed a popular expository pulpit style characterized by a clear and accurate presentation of Scripture, with a marked emphasis on the practical application of the Bible to everyday living, making God's truths a reality in the lives of hurting people.

Raised in Houston, Texas, and having originally pursued a career in engineering, Dr. Swindoll entered Dallas Theological Seminary in 1959 and graduated four years later with honors. In June 1977 an honorary doctor of divinity degree was conferred on him by Talbot Theological Seminary in La Mirada, California.

Since 1971 Dr. Swindoll has been senior pastor at the First Evangelical Free Church of Fullerton, California.

Currently, Dr. Swindoll's ministry is shared internationally through an extensive cassette tape distribution and a thirty-minute daily radio broadcast—"Insight for Living"—now being aired more than seven hundred times each day worldwide. "Insight for Living" received the prestigious Award of Merit from National

Religious Broadcasters for the outstanding religious broadcast in 1982.

A growing list of Dr. Swindoll's published works include the Christian film, *People of Refuge;* a six-message film series, *Strengthening Your Grip;* and more than fourteen books, among which are *Dropping Your Guard; Strengthening Your Grip; Improving Your Serve; Strike the Original Match;* and *Three Steps Forward, Two Steps Back.* Also available are sixteen booklets: *Anger, Attitudes, Commitment, Demonism, Destiny, Divorce, Eternal Security, God's Will, Hope, Integrity, Leisure, Sensuality, Singleness, Stress, Tongues,* and *Woman.*

Dr. Swindoll and his wife, Cynthia, have four children—Curtis and Charissa (both married) and Colleen and Chuck (both students still living at home). The Swindolls reside in Fullerton, California.

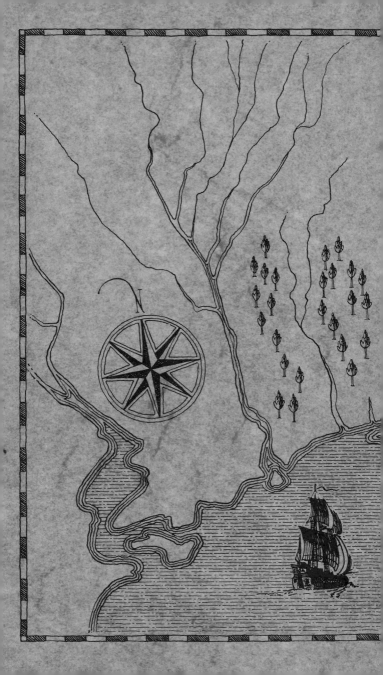